Paleo Tacos

50 Healthy, Scrumptious and Easy to make Paleo Recipes

Disclaimer

The author has tried to be an authentic source of the information provided in this report. However, the author does not oppose the additional information available over the internet. The objective of providing different Paleolithic recipes is to enable readers to try these delicious recipes at home. The recipes of Paleo food included in this book cannot be compared with the preparation methods of the same provided in other books. All readers can seek further help through additional sources of information.

Ignoring any of the guidelines or not following each step of the preparation method of Paleo dishes may not give you the exact result. Therefore, the author is not responsible for such negligence.

Contents

Why You Should Adopt Paleo Diet?

Paleo diet only sounds like a non appetizing idea but it is not! The Paleo recipes are easy, quick and to top all healthy. They are easy on budget and economical.

Paleo food keeps your body healthy and reduces the risk of heart diseases, high/low blood pressure and other dangerous diseases like diabetes. They say prevention is better than cure. Paleo diet is the easy way to prevent the diseases and other health related problems.

They also help you in losing weight and make you active and healthy in your daily tasks and routines. It improves your digestion. So just go ahead and try a Paleo diet.

Recipe: World's Best SOFT Shell Taco recipe the Paleo way

Soft Shell Taco:

Serving: 2-3 Persons

Cooking Time: 20 Minutes

Ingredients:

Half cup of Almond flour

Half cup arrowroot powder

4 eggs (Yolk removed, whisked)

2 tablespoon of water

Salt according to taste

Pepper according to taste

Coconut Oil, according to need

Process:

Take a bowl and add almond flour, arrowroot powder, egg whites, water, salt and pepper. Mix them together and form a batter. Now place a pan on stove and pour one teaspoon of coconut oil on it. Grease the pan and pour the batter in the center spread it round in a circle, slowly. It will look like a thin pancake. Change sides and cook for 30 - 40 seconds.

Allow the taco to be cooled down enjoy it with you favorite Paleo filling!

Recipe: World's Best HARD Shell Taco recipe the Paleo way

Soft Shell Taco:

Serving: 2-3 Persons

Cooking Time: 20 Minutes

Ingredients:

4 tablespoon of coconut flour

4 tablespoon of flax seed (crushed to powder)

1 cup of milk (coconut milk)

Mexican herbs and spices to taste

Process:

Heat an oven at 400F. In the meanwhile take a bowl and add all the ingredients mix them all well together and knead to form dough. The dough will be relatively stiff and thick. Take small portions and roll them out in round circles. Take any cylindrical object and place the taco on it. You can even use the muffin baking tray. Turn it upside down and place the rolled out taco sheets in the center. Now place the muffin baking tray inside the preheated oven. Bake the tacos for 20 minutes. Serve hot or cold, fill the hard taco shells with your favorite Paleo filling and enjoy!

Scrumptious Paleo Taco Recipes

Taco with Fruit Salsa

Serving: 6 persons

Cooking Time: 10 minutes

Ingredients:

6 homemade Paleo hard taco shells

1 cup tomatoes, cut into small cubes

1.5 teaspoon of kosher salt

¼ teaspoon Black pepper, freshly crushed

½ cup of red onion chopped nicely

1cup mango, cut into cubes

1/2 cup of pineapple, cut into small cubes

1.5 jalapenos, seeds removed, cut into small cubes

4 cloves of garlic, coarsely chopped

1 cup of cilantro leaves, coarsely chopped

4 tablespoon of lime juice

3 teaspoons of olive oil

Process:

Take a bowl and add tomato, kosher salt, Black pepper, red onion mango, pineapple, jalapenos, garlic, cilantro leaves, lime juice and olive oil. Mix all the ingredients gently with help of a fork. Take hard taco shells and fill the center with the fruit salsa. Serve immediately.

Taco with Apple Tikka

Serving: 10 Persons

Cooking Time: 45 Minutes

Ingredients:

2 tablespoon of red chili powder

1 tablespoon of oregano crushed

2Tablespoon of coconut flour

2 tablespoon of flaxseed meal

Salt to taste

Pepper to taste

Turmeric powder, half teaspoon

Half teaspoon of nutmeg powder

3 tablespoon olive oil

2 cups of apple, cut in 1 inch cubes

5-6 soft taco shells

Process:

Take a bowl and add all the ingredients in it except taco shell. Now mix all the ingredients together and place aside to marinade the apples. Now take skewers and place the apple cubes on it. In a grilling pan add oil and when it is ready place the apple skewers in it. Cook from each side for 4 minutes and then turn. When ready take the apples off of the skewers and place them on soft taco shells. Serve immediately. Enjoy!

Taco with Spicy Beef

Serving: 10-12 Persons

Cooking Time: 1.5 Hours

Ingredients:

12 hard Shell tacos

2 lbs beef roast cut into strips;

1 cup of mushrooms;

1 cup of green onions,

1 cup beef stock

0.5cup coconut milk;

0.5 cup white wine

1 tsp mustard

Olive oil

Sea salt

Pepper to taste

Process:

Take a bowl and add strips of beef in it. Season the strips with salt and pepper. In the meanwhile, take a pan and heat oil in it. Add the beef strips and allow them to get a bit tender. After 5-8 minutes add green onions and other vegetables and sauté them for 5 minutes. Don't stir too much. Add the white wine and allow the mixture to come to boil. Place a lid on the pan and cook for 5 minutes to allow the beef to get tender. When all the liquid in the pan get s dried or when most of it has been dried off, add the beef stock. Now allow the mixture to come to boil again. Cook for (50 minutes) let the sauce get a bit thick, check for seasoning. Place the beef and a bit of sauce in the hard shell taco and serve immediately.

Taco with Miniature Meat Balls

Serving: 5 persons

Cooking Time: 1 Hour

Ingredients:

10-15 Home made Paleo Hard Shell Tacos

2 pounds of lean beef;

Half a cup of cup green onions, chopped

Half a cup of cup almond flour

1 egg, (whisked)

Half a teaspoon of chili powder

Coconut oil, according to need

Sea salt according to taste

Black pepper, freshly crushed

For the Meat ball sauce:

2 tablespoon of apple cider vinegar

1 cup ketchup (homemade)

½ up of finely chopped onion

¼ tablespoon of paprika;

2 tablespoon of coconut aminos

Sea salt according to taste

Black pepper, freshly crushed

¼ tablespoon of chili powder

Process:

Heat an oven at 400F. In the meanwhile, take a bowl and mix all the ingredients other than of the sauce. Mix all the ingredients and knead them to make it appear of uniform consistency. If the mixture gets a bit dry, add 2-3 tablespoon of water and knead for 2-3 minutes. Now take the mixture and form small nature meatballs. Place them aside. Take baking dray grease it with oil and then place the tray in the pre heated oven.

In the mean while prepare the sauce for the meat balls. Take a large skillet and add all the ingredients for sauce and stir well until it is boiling. Check for salt and pepper and cook for 5 more minutes or until it is thick like ketchup.

Take out the meat balls from the oven and add them to the sauce. Stir well make sure you don't break the meat balls. Now take the tacos and add meat balls in the center with the BBQ sauce and roll it. Secure with tooth pick. Serve hot.

Taco with Roast beef (Balsamic)

Serving: 10 People

Cooking Time: 2.5 Hours

Ingredients:

10-12 Taco Shell (Hard/Soft, your choice)

1.3 Kg boneless beef

2 cups of sweet potatoes, (Cut into squares)

1.5 cup of carrots, (Cut into slices)

Half cup of Onion, diced

1/8 tsp of rosemary

Bay leaves 2-3

1 tablespoon of garlic, chopped coarsely

1/2 cup balsamic vinegar;

1 ½ cup of vegetable stock

2 tbsp walnut oil

1 cup white wine

Black pepper to taste

Sea salt to taste

***Process*:**

Take a bowl and add strips of beef in it. Season the beef with salt and pepper. In the meanwhile, take a pan and heat oil in it. Add the beef and allow it to get brown on both sides. Now add the beef stock, garlic, bay leaves, onion and vinegar in the pan and stir well. Allow the mixture to come to boil and beef to get a bit tender.

After 5-8 minutes add carrots and sweet potatoes, sauté them for 5 minutes. Don't stir too much. Add the white wine and allow the mixture to come to boil. Place a lid on the pan and cook for 1-2 hours to allow the beef to get tender. When all the liquid in the pan gets dried or when the beef is fork tender. Take the roast out of the pot and cut it into slices or into chunks. Take a bowl add the chunks and the vegetables. Check for seasoning and then add the mixture to the tacos and serve hot.

Taco with Beef Salad

Serving: 10-12 Persons

Cooking Time: 30 Minutes

Ingredients:

10-12 Tacos (Soft or Hard shell)

0.5 Kg beef, cut into strips

2-3 tablespoon of Avocado or Olive oil (to brown the beef)

Sea salt to taste

Pepper to taste

For Salad Dressing:

3 cups of broccoli florets

4 cups of salad greens

2 cups of spring onion

1 cup of Baby tomatoes, Cut into square

Half a cup of red and yellow capsicum, Juliana cut

1 cup onion, cut into slices

2/3 cup of vinaigrette

Process:

Take a bowl and add strips of beef in it. Season the beef with salt and pepper. In the meanwhile, take a pan and heat oil in it. Add the beef and allow it to get brown. In the mean while prepare the salad dressing. Add all the ingredients in a large bowl and toss them together except for vinaigrette and broccoli. Place a pan on stove and add the vinaigrette in it. Allow it to get a bit warm and then add the broccoli in it. Stir a bit and allow the mixture to come to boil.

Now add the strips of beef in the pan and stir well. After 5-10 minutes remove the pan from stove and add beef and broccoli mixture in the bowl of vegetables and mix all the ingredients with fork. Place the mixture in taco of your choice and serve.

Tacos with Tip Roast

Serving: Serves 6-7

Cooking Time: 2 Hours

Ingredients:

10-12 Tacos (Soft or Hard shell)

Kg of round trip roast

Black pepper to taste

Sea salt to taste;

1.5 tablespoon of garlic, coarsely chopped

1 tablespoon of dried oregano

1 Tablespoon of basil (dried and crushed)

1 tablespoon of red pepper flakes

Coconut oil for cooking

Process:

Heat the oven at 250-300F for baking. Now take a bowl, and mix basil, garlic, salt, pepper and red pepper flakes. Place the roast in a large baking tray and rub the mixture of spices on all the sides. Rib well and cover all of it.

In the mean while take a large pot and some oil in it. Place the roast in the pan and brown it from all the sides. Place the beef on the baking tray. Make sure you place a grill on the pan and then place the beef on it. Place the roast in the oven for 1.5 hours. Check the beef after an hour to see how much is done. Take the beef out and then cut into slices. Shred the slices into strips and serve with your choice of tacos.

Tacos with Asada Sirloin

Serving: 10-12 Persons

Cooking Time: 3 Hours

Ingredients:

10-12 Soft or Hard Shell tacos

1.5 Kg steak

1 tablespoon of chopped garlic

0.5 tablespoon of oregano (dried and crushed)

1 tablespoon of paprika or crushed red pepper

1 tablespoon of chili powder

½ tsp. cumin

2 tablespoon of lemon juice (fresh)

Black pepper to taste;

Sea salt to taste;

Process:

Take a bowl and add the spices, salt, pepper, red crushed pepper, oregano, and garlic. Mix well. Place a meat in a large bowel pour the lemon on it. Rub the lemon on its surface well. Now sprinkle the season prepared on the meat and rub them on the meat well 1 hour minutes. Keep the meat aside allow the meat to absorb the flavors of the spices and seasoning.

Take a large skillet and add some oil in its place the meat in the pan and allow it to cook from both sides. Cook until it is according to your liking. Take out the meat and then cut it into strips. Check for seasoning and then serve with tacos of your choice.

Tacos with Cuban chicken and vegetables

**Serving:** 5-6 People

**Cooking Time:**

All together 8 hours

**Ingredients:**

5-6 Tacos (Soft or Hard shell)

1 kg beef chuck (ground and lean)

1.5 tablespoon of garlic, coarsely chopped

1 cup of onion, Juliana cut

Half teaspoon of cumin

2 tablespoon of orange juice

½ tablespoon of lime zest

2 tablespoon of lime juice

1 cup of beef /chicken or vegetable stock

Black pepper to taste

Sea salt to taste

Olive Oil

**Process:**

Take a bowl and add beef chuck in it and Season with salt and pepper. Rub the salt and pepper seasoning on its surface well. Put the seasoned beef in a large skillet and add the stock in it, Cover the lid and allow the roast to get tender, cook for approximately 4-hours. When the beef is done cut it into pieces or chunks as you like it.

Take a felt and add olive oil in it. Place the garlic and onion in the pan fry them until garlic is fragrant. Now add the beef in the skillet and toss it well. Allow the beef to get a bit fried and then sprinkle the lemon zest and pour in the orange juice. Mix all the ingredients and allow them to come to a bowl. Add the cumin powder in the mixture and stir well. When all of the liquid is dry and thick, serve it with tacos of your choice.

Tacos with zucchini and chicken salad

Serving: 5-6 Persons

Cooking Time: 30 Minutes

Ingredients:

10-12 Tacos (Soft or Hard shell)

0.5 Kg boneless chicken

2-3 tablespoon of Avocado or Olive oil (to brown the beef)

Sea salt to taste

Pepper to taste

1 tablespoon of chili powder;

2 cups grapes

1 cup blueberries;

3 cups lettuce cut into pieces

Half cup Zucchini cut into thin strips

4 tablespoon full of almonds crushed

Olive Oil

Sea salt to taste

Pepper to taste

Salad Dressing

3 tablespoon of almond butter

2 tablespoon of orange juice

3 tablespoon of water

1 tablespoon of mustard

½ tablespoon of honey

½ garlic, coarsely chopped

Sea salt to taste

Process:

Take a bowl and add chunk of chicken in it. Season it with salt and pepper. In the meanwhile, take a pan and heat oil in it. Add the chicken and allow it to get brown. In the mean while prepare the salad dressing. Add all the ingredients in a large skillet and put it over heat. Keep whisking the ingredients. Now take a bowl and add all the fruits and green vegetables in it. Add chicken and drizzle the almond dressing over it. Sprinkle the crushed almonds and season the salad with spices, salt and pepper. Mix all the ingredients with fork. Place the mixture in taco of your choice and serve.

Tacos with Chicken and Apricots

**Serving:** 10-12 Persons

**Cooking Time:** 30 Minutes

**Ingredients:**

10-12 Tacos

1lb chicken, boneless cut into bite sized pieces

3 tablespoon walnut oil

Sea salt & Pepper for seasoning

1 cup of onions cut into cubes

4 cups of collard greens

1 cup of red berries

2 cup of Apricots

1 + 2 tablespoon of lemon juice

2 cups of lettuce

Half a cup of capsicum, Juliana cut

**Process**:

Take a bowl and add strips of chicken in it. Season it with salt and pepper and 1 tablespoon of lemon juice. Take a pan and heat oil in it. Add the chicken and brown it. Add all the vegetables and fruits in the bowl and toss them together. Add lemon juice and mix well. Now add the strips of chicken in the bowl and mix well. Place the mixture in taco of your choice and serve.

Tacos with Prosciutto wraps

Serving: 5-6 persons

Cooking Time: 30 Minutes

Ingredients:

5-6 Tacos (Soft or Hard shell)

0.5 kg chicken cube, 1/2 inch (boneless)

0.25 kg prosciutto

1 cup onion (chopped coarsely)

Half a cup of vegetable stock

1 tablespoon of mustard (grounded)

2 tablespoon of Coconut milk

2 tablespoon of parsley chopped

1 tablespoon of Olive Oil

Black pepper to taste

Process:

Take a bowl and add the chicken cubes in it. Add mustard, salt and pepper in it and mix well. Cover all the chicken pieces with the spices and put the aside. Take the prosciutto wraps and place one chicken cube, and wrap the prosciuttos around it. Repeat the procedure with all the cubes. Now take a skillet and add 5-6 tablespoon of olive oil in it. Now add all the wraps in it and fry them. Fry the prosciutto wraps until they are golden brown or crisp. Make sure you cook them on medium heat so that chicken cubes can get nicely done.

Take out the wraps and then add the onion, vegetable stock, parsley in the pan and sauté them over medium or low heat. Add the coconut milk and stir on low heat. When the mixture is thick and ready drizzle it over the chicken wraps and coat them nicely. Serve with your favorite tacos.

Tacos with mushroom and chicken sauce

__Serving:__ 5-6 Persons

__Cooking Time:__ 2 Hour

__Ingredients:__

5-6 hard Shell tacos

1 cup of mushrooms, (Thinly sliced)

1 cup chicken stock

1 kg chicken cut into strips

1 cup coconut milk;

1 cup of green collards (boiled),

0.5 cup balsamic vinegar

1 teaspoon of grounded mustard powder

5-6 Tablespoon of Avocado Oil

Sea salt to taste

Pepper to taste

__Process__:

Take a bowl and add strips of chicken in it. Season the strips with salt and pepper. In the meanwhile, take a pan and heat oil in it. Add the chicken strips and allow them to get a bit tender. After 5-8 minutes add green collards and other vegetables and sauté them for 5 minutes. Add the balsamic vinegar and allow the mixture to come to boil.

Place a lid on the pan and cook for 10 minutes to allow the chicken to get tender. When all the liquid in the pan get s dried or when most of it has been dried off, add the chicken stock. Cook for 50 minutes, let the sauce get a bit thick, check for seasoning. Place the chicken and a bit of sauce in the taco shell (of your choice) and serve immediately.

Tacos with Avocado Salad

Serving: 8-10 Persons

Cooking Time: 25 Minutes

Ingredients:

1 Kg Boneless Chicken (cut into small cubes ort strips)

1.5 cup of avocado (cut into small cubes)

1 teaspoon of garlic, coarsely chopped

1 cup red bell pepper, (cut into cubes)

1 cup of celery, (cut into cubes)

Half a cup of green onions, finely chopped

6 tablespoon of olive oil

2 tablespoon of lemon juice

Sea salt to taste

Pepper, to taste

Process:

Take a large skillet and add2-3 tablespoon of olive oil in it. When the oil is heated up add garlic and sauté over medium heat until fragrant. Now add the chicken cubes in the skillet and stir well. Cook the chicken cubes until they are no longer pink.

Add the capsicum in this skillet and stir well not cook too much they should be crunchy while serving with tacos. Check for seasoning and add the salt and pepper according to your taste. Take out the chicken and capsicum and add 2 tablespoon of oil in the skillet. Add the avocados, green onions; lemon juice, chopped celery and sauté them toss until all the vegetables are evenly coated with olive oil. Cook the vegetables for 3-4 minutes and then add the chicken in the skillet. Mix well and take it out in a bowl. Serve with the tacos shell of your choice.

Taco Pie

Serving: 8 persons

Cooking Time: 2 hours

Ingredients:

6-7 Soft shell tacos

0.25 Kg. Chicken cubes, (Boiled and cooked)

0.25 lbs beef cut into strips (fried and cooked in oil, seasoned)

1 cup of onion (Juliana Cut)

2 Cups of Carrots (Cut into cubes)

1 leek, (Cut into cubes);

4 cups tomatoes (Cut into cubes)

1 cup vegetable stock

1 tablespoon of homemade Worcestershire sauce (optional)

Avocado Cooking Oil

Freshly crushed black pepper, to taste

Sea salt to taste

For Sweet potato layer:

1 kg sweet potatoes, (peeled, boiled and cut into cubes)

Half cup of clarified butter

Black pepper, to taste

Sea salt to taste

Process:

Heat the oven at 370F. Take the boiled mash potatoes and cut them into small cubes. Put them aside. In the mean while take a skillet and add olive oil or Avocado oil in it. And brown the beef strips in it. When they are cooked take them out of the skillet and put them aside.

Now in the skillet add the clarified butter and add the mashed and boiled sweet potatoes in it. Mix them well and season with salt and pepper according to your taste. You can add parsley to enhance the taste of the mashed sweet potatoes.

Take another skillet and add the olive oil in it. Add tomatoes and allow them to get a bit tender. Now add the vegetables stock in the pan and stir well. Allow the tomatoes to get completely soft in the broth. Add the home made Worcestershire sauce and stir well. Allow the mixture to come to boil. Add the beef strips and chicken cubes in the mixture and cook for about 20 minutes. Pour the mixture in a baking tray. Place the soft actor she on top of it. Don't press and place the layers. Not spread the mashed potatoes on top. And cover completely. Place the baking tray inside the oven and bake for 30 minutes. Take out cut into pieces and serve hot.

Tacos with Beef Satay

Serving:

Cooking Time:

Ingredients:

For sauce:

Half cup of cup almond butter or clarified butter

1 minced shallot

1 teaspoon of ginger, coarsely chopped

1 teaspoon of chopped lemongrass

Half cup of coconut milk;

1 teaspoon of Olive Oil

Black pepper to taste

Sea salt to taste

For Satay:

1 Kg beef cut into strips

2 minced shallot

1 tablespoon of coarsely chopped garlic,

2 red chilies cut into pieces

1 tablespoon of fresh ginger, minced;

Half a tablespoon of lemongrass

3 tablespoon of coconut milk

2 tablespoon of fish sauce

4 tablespoon of honey (raw)

2 tablespoon of olive oil;

Process:

Take a bowl and add the beef trips in it and add all the spices and other ingredients for the stay and mix well. Coat all the strips together and well. Put it aside for an hour or so for marinating. Now take a skillet and the olive oil or clarified butter in it. Add the lemon grass, ginger and salt in it add the shallot pieces and stir well. Cook until they are crisp golden. Pour in the coconut milk in the skillet and add the almond butter and salt. Stir well and allow the mixture to come to boil.

Take skewers and place the marinated beef on it. Grill the beef until it is cooked and pour the butter sauce on it. Serve with your favorite taco shell.

Tacos with grilled chicken salad

Serving: 8-10 Persons

Cooking Time: 30 Minutes

Ingredients:

1 Kg Boneless Chicken (cut into small cubes or to be easily placed on skewers)

1 teaspoon of garlic, coarsely chopped

1 cup red and green bell pepper, Juliana cut

2cups of Lettuce, (torn into pieces)

1 cup of celery, (cut into cubes)

1 cup of collard green, (boiled)

1 cup of green onions, finely chopped

2 tablespoon of raw honey (Mixed in ¼ cup of water for drizzling)

Half cup of baby tomatoes

6 tablespoon of olive oil

2 tablespoon of lemon juice

Sea salt to taste

Pepper, to taste

Process:

Take a large skillet and add 2-3 tablespoon of olive oil in it. When the oil is heated up add garlic and sauté over medium heat until fragrant. Now add the chicken cubes in the skillet and stir well. Add the bell pepper in this skillet and stir well, do not overcook. Check for seasoning and add the salt and pepper.

Take out the chicken and bell pepper and add tablespoon of oil in the skillet. Add the lettuce, green onions, collard greens, lemon juice, chopped celery, and sauté them toss until all the vegetables are evenly coated with olive oil. Cook the vegetables for 3-4 minutes and then add the chicken in the skillet. Mix well and take it out in a bowl Drizzle the honey and water syrup. Serve with the tacos shell of your choice.

Tacos with Mango and Chicken Salad

Serving: 5-6 Persons

Cooking Time: 30 Minutes

Ingredients:

10-12 Tacos (Soft or Hard shell)

0.5 Kg boneless chicken

3 tablespoon +3 tablespoon of Olive oil (to brown the chicken)

1 tablespoon of chili powder;

2 cups grapes

1 cup baby tomatoes;

Half a cup of boiled sprouts

1 Cup of Mangoes (Cut into cubes)

3 cups lettuce cut into pieces

Olive Oil

Sea salt to taste

Pepper to taste

2 tablespoon of lemon juice

1 tablespoon of mustard

½ tablespoon of raw honey

½ garlic, coarsely chopped

Process:

Take a bowl and add chunk of chicken in it. Season it with salt and pepper. In the meanwhile, take a pan and heat oil in it. Add the chicken and allow it to get brown. Add 3tablespoons of Olive oil in a large skillet add the garlic in it and sauté until fragrant. Add the baby tomatoes, sprouts, collard greens chili powder, lemon juice, mustard, salt and pepper and mix all the ingredients well.

Take a bowl and add mangoes, grapes in it. Put all the vegetables in a bowl and add the chicken in it. Mix gently and serve with tacos of your choice and serve.

Tacos with Honey Mustard Chicken

Serving: 5-6

Cooking Time: 40 Minutes

Ingredients:

6 taco shells (soft or hard)

1 Kg boneless chicken (cut into cubes)

5-6 Taco shells (Soft or Hard)

4 tablespoon of raw honey

4 tablespoon of brown mustard (spicy)

Half a tablespoon of lemon juice

Sea salt to taste

Ground pepper to taste

Process:

Heat the oven at 350-400F. In the meanwhile steam the chicken in the broiler and put it aside. Place steamed chicken pieces to refrigerate for 20-30 minutes. Take them out and place them in the baking tray over a baking rack. Place the tray inside the oven and bake the chicken until the crust is a bit golden brown in color.

In the meanwhile, in a large bowl add the salt, pepper, lemon juice, mustard and honey mix all the ingredients well. Whisk until the mixture is of uniform consistency. Pour the mixture in a skillet and place it over the stove. Allow the mixture to come to a mild boiling temperature. Take out the chicken pieces from the oven and place it in a bowl. Dip all the pieces in the honey mustard mixture and place them back on the baking tray. Place the tray in the oven and bake for another 20 minutes. Serve the chicken with your favorite tacos.

Tacos with thyme Chicken

Serving: 5 Persons

Cooking Time: 50 Minutes

Ingredients:

5 taco shells (soft or hard)

4 chicken breasts

3 tablespoon of garlic, chopped coarsely

½ cup of vegetable stock

1 teaspoon full of lemon zest

¼ cup of lemon juice

3 sprigs of thyme

Sea salt to taste

Ground pepper to taste

Process:

Heat the oven at 350-400F. In the meanwhile, place the chicken breast in a tray and sprinkle salt and pepper on them. Sprinkle the seasoning on both sides. Now take a baking tray and place the chicken breast on them and add the garlic, thyme sprigs, broth, and lemon zest in the tray.

Place the tray inside the pre-heated oven and bake the chicken for 40 minutes. Change the sides carefully, not breaking the breast. Take out the chicken and cut into stripes. Serve with your favorite taco shell (soft or hard).

Tacos with chicken Tikka

Serving: 10 Persons

Cooking Time: 1.5 hours

Ingredients:

2 tablespoon of red chili powder

1 Tablespoon of Mustard Powder

1 tablespoon of oregano crushed

2 Tablespoon of coconut flour

2 tablespoon of flaxseed meal

4tablespoon of coconut milk

Salt to taste

Pepper to taste

Turmeric powder, half teaspoon

Half teaspoon of nutmeg powder

3 tablespoon olive oil

1 kg of chicken boneless, cut into cubes (to be placed on skewers)

10 taco shells (soft or hard)

Process:

Take a bowl and add all the ingredients in it except taco shell. Now mix all the ingredients together and place aside to marinade the chicken for approx 1 hour. Now take skewers and place the chicken on it.

Heat the grill and place the chicken skewers on it. Cook from each side for 5-8 minutes and then turn. When ready take the chicken Tikka off of the skewers and place them on taco shells. Serve immediately.

Tacos with turkey Chili

Serving: 5 Persons

Cooking Time: 1 Hour

Ingredients:

5-6 taco shells (soft or hard)

1 lbs of turkey meat (Boiled, cooked and shredded)

2 cups of thinly sliced carrots

2 cups of chopped onions (half inch pieces),

1 cup of capsicum (Cut into thin strips, Juliana cut),

2 cups of tomatoes, (Cut into thin strips, Juliana cut),

2 tablespoon of tomato paste

1.5 tablespoon of minced garlic

1 cup chicken broth

2 tablespoon of chili powder or to taste

1 tablespoon of ground cumin;

1 tablespoon of flakes of red pepper

1 tablespoon of oregano (crushed)

Avocado oil

Sea salt to taste

Black pepper to taste;

Green onions, sliced (optional, for garnishing);

Process:

Take a pan and add avocado oil in it. Only enough to sauté chopped onions in it. Keep stirring, allow the onions to get a bit golden brown and then add sliced carrots, capsicum it. Sauté the vegetables for 5 minutes and then add the spices in it and mix all the ingredients well. Add the diced tomatoes and turkey in the pan and stir well. Adjust the salt and paper according to your taste.

Now pour in the chicken broth and allow the mixture to come to boil. When the mixture is reduced to half take it out in a bowl and serve with your favorite tacos.

Tacos with Chicken and Zucchini Noodles

Serving: 10 Persons

Cooking Time: 30 Minutes

Ingredients:

10-12 Tacos (Soft or Hard shell)

1 lbs of Zucchini noodles

0.5 Kg boneless chicken (boiled)

2-3 tablespoon of Olive oil (to brown the chicken)

1 tablespoon of lemon juice

1Tablepsoon of Paprika

1 Cup of baby tomatoes

Sea salt to taste

Pepper to taste

1 tablespoon of chili powder;

½ garlic, coarsely chopped

Process:

Take a pan and heat oil in it. Take a bowl and add chunk of boiled chicken in it. Season it with salt and pepper. Add the chicken in the pan on stove and allow it to get brown. In the meanwhile, boil the zucchini noodles, drain them and put them aside.

In a frying pan add 2 tablespoon of olive oil, salt and paper. Add zucchini noodles in it and fry for 2 minutes and then add baby tomatoes chicken and lemon juice. Sauté them well and take them out in plate. Serve with your favorite taco as filling. Enjoy!

Tacos with creamy chicken and squash

Serving: 5 Persons

Cooking Time: 1 Hours

Ingredients:

5 Tacos (Soft or Hard shell)

3 cups of squash, removed seeds and cut into small cubes

1 kg of Chicken (boneless, cut into small cubes)

0.5 Kg of Mushrooms cut into slices (Button mushroom)

Half a cup of Onions, (Chopped into small cubes)

1 cup of carrot, (cut into thin slices)

2 celery stalks, (cut into small cubes)

2 tablespoon of Olive oil or any other Paleo nut oil

2 tablespoon of minced garlic

12 oz coconut milk

5 tablespoon of parsley, coarsely chopped

Sea salt to taste

Pepper to taste

Process:

Heat the oven at 350-370F. Spray the olive oil on the squash and marinate them with salt and pepper according to your taste. Take a baking tray. Slightly grease it and then place all the squash pieces in it. Place the tray inside the oven for 20-25 minutes and allow the squashes to get a roasted a bit.

In the mean while place a pan on the stove and add olive oil in it and add the garlic in it, when the garlic is fragrant, add onions and sauté them until they are translucent. Add rest of the vegetables in the pan and sauté them. Don't overcook the vegetables; they should be a little crispy.

Now add the chicken and cook them over low heat. Add the mushrooms stir a bit and pour in the coconut milk in the pan. Adjust the salt and pepper and stir a little. Take out the squash from the oven and mash it. Add the squash in the pan and mix. When the mixture is a bit thick take it out in a bowl. Serve with your favorite taco as filling. Enjoy!

Tacos with baked chicken nuggets

Serving: 5 persons

Cooking Time: 30 Minutes

Ingredients:

5 Tacos (Soft or Hard shell)

1 kg Chicken (boneless)

2 eggs (whisked)

3 cups of almond flour

1 teaspoon of garlic powder

1 teaspoon of paprika

1 teaspoon of dried oregano

Sea salt to taste

Pepper to taste

Thick Sauce:

1 cup of homemade mayo

1 tablespoon of minced garlic

1 tablespoon of minced chives

Sea salt to taste

Pepper to taste

Process:

Heat the oven at 370 – 400 F. in the meanwhile Take the chicken breasts and flatten them with help of a plastic hammer. And cut them into 1 inch cubes to make nuggets. Put the chicken aside. Take another bowl and add all the dry ingredients like salt and pepper, flour, paprika, garlic powder and oregano in it. Mix all the ingredients well.

Take another bowl and pour in the whisked eggs in it. Take one piece of chicken and coat it well in the whisked eggs and coat it with the flour mixture e and place it in a plate. Repeat the procedure with all of the chicken pieces. Place the coated chicken pieces in the fridge to settle down a bit. Then take them out and place them on the greased baking tray. Put the baking tray inside the oven and cook for 15 minutes and turn them over and bake them for another 15 minutes. In the mean while prepare a thick sauce for the nuggets.

Mix the sauce ingredients in a bowl and whisk well. Take the tacos shells (preferably soft shell) and spread the thick sauce all over them. Place the chicken baked nuggets ion it. Roll over and serve hot.

Tacos with chicken and artichokes

Serving: 7-8 Persons

Cooking Time: 30 Minutes

Ingredients:

7-8 tacos

0.4 KG of boneless chicken (cut into thin strips and cooked)

2 cups cut into pieces artichoke

2 cup of tomatoes (cut into thin strips, Juliana cut)

1 cup of black and green olives, cut into slices

¾ cup fresh basil, chopped

1.5 cup olive oil

2 tablespoon of white vinegar

1 tablespoon of lemon juice

Sea salt to taste

Pepper to taste

Process:

Heat a grill for grilling. Take a bowl and add artichokes in it. Pour some olive oil on it and toss them well. Put the artichokes on the grill and grill them for good 2-3 minutes. Take them off of the grill.

In a bowl add the tomatoes olives and chicken and mix them well. In another bowl mix Olive oil, white vinegar, lemon juice and adjust the salt and pepper. Add the grilled artichokes with the chicken and other vegetables and drizzle the olive and vinegar mixture on top. Toss the salad together and serve with your favorite tacos

Tacos with mushroom and chicken sauce

Serving: 5 persons

Cooking Time: 1 hour

Ingredients:

1 Kg of Chicken boneless, Cut into 2 inch strips

1 cup of minced shallot

1 cup of button mushrooms, cut into thin slices

2 tablespoon of minced chives

Half a cup of chicken broth (you can even use the vegetable stock)

4 tablespoon of coconut milk

1 tablespoon of Avocado Oil

Sea salt to taste

Pepper to taste

Process:

Heat the oven at 300 – 350F. Take the chicken and place it in a greased baking tray and place it inside the preheated oven for about 30-40 minutes. Take out the chicken when it is done.

Place a large skillet on the stove and heat some oil in it. Add the shallots in the skillet and cook them for about 2-3 minutes then add the mushroom slices and stir well. Add the chicken or vegetable broth. Mix all the ingredients well. Pour in the coconut milk and cook until the mixture is a bit thick. In the meanwhile, take out the chicken and add the baked chicken in the sauce. Take it out and serve the chicken with thick hot gravy with soft taco shell. .

Tacos with lemon chicken Kebabs

Serving Size: 4-6 Person

Cooking Time: 50 Minutes

Ingredients:

5 Tacos (Soft or Hard shell)

1 lb minced chicken meat

0.25 cup of lemon juice

Pinch of Cardamom

2 tablespoon of lemon zest

Half cup of chopped onion

1 ½ teaspoon of Cinnamon

2 tablespoon of Cilantro

¾ teaspoon of Ginger

Sea salt to taste

Pepper to taste

¾ tablespoon of nutmeg

1 tablespoon of Raw Honey

Process

Heat a grill. Take a bowl and add nutmeg, ginger, salt, pepper, cardamom, lemon zest and cinnamon. Now add the chicken mince in the bowl along with onion, honey and cilantro. Mix all the ingredients well with help of hands. Knead the mixture. Now take the iron skewers and apply the mixture in form of small kebabs on the skewers. Place the skewers on the preheated grill and drizzle a bit of olive oil. Cook the kebabs from both sides and take them off. Serve with your favorite taco shell.

Tacos with roasted vegetables

Serving: 10 Persons

Cooking Time: 30 Minutes

Ingredients:

10-12 Tacos (Soft or Hard shell)

2-3 tablespoon of Avocado

Sea salt to taste

Pepper to taste

1 tablespoon of Paprika

3 cups lettuce torn into pieces

Half cup Zucchini cut into thin slices

1 Cup of Onions cut into strips

1 cup of Tomatoes cut into strips, seeds removed

1 Cup of capsicum, cut into strips

2 tablespoon of orange juice

Process:

Heat a grill pan and place all the vegetables on it. Keep tossing them after every 30 seconds. Toast the vegetables for about 5 minutes and then drizzle one tablespoon of olive oil on it. And stir the vegetables. Cook for another 2 minutes and then sprinkle paprika and salt over it. Drizzle rest of the olive oil and, lemon juice on the vegetables and toss them Adjust the salt and pepper and take them out of the pan. Serve with your favorite taco shell.

Tacos with Chicken Asparagus Carbonara

Serving: 7-8 Persons

Cooking Time: 30 minutes

Ingredients:

8 taco shells (Hard or soft according to your choice)

1 bowl of squash spaghetti

0.5 Kg of chicken (boneless, cut into cubes)

2 cups of cubes of asparagus pieces;

Half cup of mushrooms cut into slices.

3 tablespoon of parsley, coarsely chopped

2 tablespoon of olive oil;

Salt and pepper for seasoning

Process:

Heat your oven at 375F for baking. Once you have prepared the spaghetti with squash, cut them in two equal halves. Take a baking tray and place the squash spaghetti on it. Spray a bit of olive oil on them and place them inside the pre heated oven for about 5-10 minutes.

In a large skillet pour in the oil, once the oil is heated up add the chicken cube sin it and sauté them until the chicken is no longer pink in color. Take the chicken out of the skillet and place it aside to cool down. Now in a deep pan add some water and add a pinch of salt in it. Add the asparagus in the pan and allow them to get cooked a bit. You can cook them until they are crispy according to your requirement.

Check on the squash spaghetti. Take them out once they are ready. Take a pan add a tablespoon of oil and brown onion and garlic in it. Add the spaghetti and asparagus and sauté them for a few minutes. Add the chicken in the pan and cook for about 2 minutes. Adjust the salt and pepper and take the carbonara out in a large dish. Fill it in the taco shell of your choice and serve immediately.

Tacos with chicken Bruschetta

Serving: Serves 4

Cooking Time: 35 Minutes

Ingredients:

4 taco shells (Hard or soft according to your choice)

0.5 kg Chicken breast (Cut into thin slices)

2 cup of tomatoes (cut into cubes)

1 cup of onion, (cut into squares)

4 tablespoon of coarsely chopped basil leaves

1 tablespoon of garlic, minced

3 tablespoon of olive oil

1 tablespoon of balsamic vinegar

Salt to taste

Black pepper to taste

2 tablespoon of paprika

1 tablespoon of oregano

Half a tablespoon of turmeric powder

1 tablespoon of raw honey

Process:

Heat the oven at 350F. In the meanwhile take a large bowl and add the vegetables in it (onions, tomatoes, chopped basil) and sprinkle the olive oil and balsamic vinegar on them and toss all the vegetable to cover them nicely in the oil and vinegar. Adjust the salt and paper according to your taste. Cover the bowl and put it aside for the vegetables to absorb the flavors.

In the meanwhile take another bow and season it with salt and pepper and all the spices and honey and mix well.

Place the pan on the stove and add oil in it. Brown the chicken until tender. Take the chicken out of the pan once it is well done and allow it to cool down a bit.

Take the tacos and place the chicken pieces on them in equal quantity. Take the bowl and place the vegetable mixture on top of the chicken. Place the taco Bruschetta on the baking tray and place them in the preheated oven to be baked for 10 minutes and then serve hot.

Tacos with cinnamon chicken

Serving: 7-8 Persons

Cooking Time: 30 Minutes

Ingredients:

7-8 tacos

0.4 KG of boneless chicken (cut into thin strips and cooked)

2/3 teaspoon of cinnamon

1 Cup chicken broth

2 cup of tomatoes (cut into thin strips, Juliana cut)

1 cup of black and green olives, cut into slices

¾ cup fresh basil, chopped

1.5 cup olive oil

2 tablespoon of white vinegar

1 tablespoon of lemon juice

Sea salt to taste

Pepper to taste

Process:

Heat a grill for grilling. Take a bowl and add artichokes in it. Pour some olive oil on it and toss them well. Put the artichokes on the grill and grill them for good 2-3 minutes. Take them off of the grill.

In a bowl add the tomatoes olives and chicken and mix them well. In another bowl mix Olive oil, white vinegar, lemon juice, cinnamon and adjust the salt and pepper. Take a pan and add a bit of oil in it. Add all the vegetables and sate them now add the grilled chicken in it and sauté for another 2-3 minutes. Pour in the chicken stock and allow the mixture to come to boil. When the liquid is reduced to less than half, drizzle the olive and vinegar mixture on top. Take your favorite tacos and fill them with the thick saucy mixture and serve hot.

Tacos with shrimp and avocado

Serving: 4 Persons

Cooking Time: 30 Minutes

Ingredients:

4 taco shells (Hard or soft according to your choice)

1 Kg raw shrimp, (cleaned and deshelled)

2 cups of mangoes, cut into cubes

1 cup avocado, cut into thin slices

1 cup tomato, cut into cubes

Half cup of cup green onions, chopped

3 tablespoon full of coarsely garlic

1 jalapeño, finely chopped

1 tablespoon of lime juice

Lemon wedges

Olive oil (according to need)

Sea salt to taste

Black pepper to taste

Process:

Take a bowl and add all the vegetables and fruits in it (green onion, mango, avocado, tomatoes) and drizzle them with lemon juice and mix all the ingredients with help of a wooden spatula. Put the bowl aside and allow the vegetables and fruits to absorb the flavor.

In the meanwhile, take a pan and add some olive oil in it. Add the shrimp once the oil in hot and sauté them for 1 minute. Sprinkle the salt and pepper from top and sauté some more. Add paprika other herbs of your choice, preferably rosemary for enhanced flavor.

When the prawns are a bit golden on top take them out. Cut the prawns into 2-3 pieces and add the pieces in the vegetable and fruit mixture. Mix well and serve with your favorite taco.

Tacos with strawberry starter

Serving: 4 Persons

Cooking Time: 35 Minutes

Ingredients:

4 taco shells (Hard or soft according to your choice)

2 cups of fresh spinach

1 cup of cooked salmon, cut into cubes (you can use chicken instead of salmon)

1 cup of strawberries, cut into slices

1 avocado, cut into thin slices

1 cup of pineapple, cut into chunks

Half a cup of onions, cut into thin slices

Half a cup of fresh pineapple juice

4 tablespoon of balsamic vinegar

1 lemon, thinly sliced

2 sprigs rosemary

1 tablespoon of olive oil

Black pepper to taste

Sea salt to taste

Process:

Heat the oven at 400 F. In the meanwhile take a baking tray and place all the lemon slices on it sprinkle the rosemary sprigs. Place the tray aside. In the mean while take another bowl and add the salmon chunks in it and season it with salt and pepper.

Sprinkle the olive oil and mix all the ingredients with rose marry and place the marinated salmon on the lemon slices in the baking tray and place the salmon in the preheated oven for about 10-20 minutes to get baked. In the meanwhile take a bowl and mix all the vegetables, strawberries, and vinegar and pineapple juice together.

Take the salmon out of the oven mix it with the vegetable mixture and serve it with your favorite taco shell.

Tacos with Thai Larb

Serving: 4 Persons

Cooking Time: 25 Minutes

Ingredients:

4 taco shells (Hard or soft according to your choice)

0.75 kg boneless chicken (cut into bite sized pieces)

0.5 cup green onions, coarsely chopped

2 tablespoon of lemongrass, coarsely chopped

2 lime leaves, chopped

1 small red chili, sliced

2 tablespoon of garlic cloves, coarsely chopped

1 tablespoon + 1 tablespoon of fish sauce

3 tablespoons olive oil

Boston lettuce leaves

Cilantro leaves

1 lime, cut into wedges

Hal f a cup fresh lemon juice

Half a teaspoon of Sriracha sauce

Process:

Blend the following ingredient until they are one, 1 tablespoon of olive oil, 1 tablespoon of fish sauce, chicken, onions, red chili, garlic lime leaves and salt and pepper according to your taste.

Blend until finely blended. In the meanwhile take a bowl and mix the remaining fish sauce, olive oil, lemon juice and Sriracha sauce. Take a pan and add a bit of olive oil allow it to get heat up. Pour in the chicken mixture in the skillet and mix well, until the chicken in the mixture changes the color to brown. When the mixture is ready take it out in a bowl and mix the chopped parsley in it. Serve with your favorite taco shells.

Tacos with orange Chicken

Serving: 5 Persons

Cooking Time: 1 Hour

Ingredients:

5-6 taco shells (soft or hard)

1 lbs of chicken (Boiled, cooked and shredded)

2 cups of thinly sliced radish

2 cups of chopped onions (half inch pieces),

2 cups of tomatoes, (Cut into thin strips, Juliana cut),

1 cup of capsicum (Cut into Juliana cut),

2 tablespoon of tomato paste

1 tablespoon of minced garlic

Half a cup of chicken stock

2 tablespoon of chili powder or to taste

1 tablespoon of flaxseed powder

1 cup of orange slices cut into pieces

Half a cup of orange juice

1 tablespoon of ground cumin;

1 tablespoon of flakes of red pepper

1 tablespoon of oregano (crushed)

Avocado oil

Sea salt to taste

Black pepper to taste;

Process:

Take a pan and add avocado oil in it. Only enough to sauté chopped onions in it. Keep stirring, allow the onions to get a bit golden brown and then add sliced radish, capsicum it. Sauté the vegetables for 5 minutes and then add the spices in it and mix all the ingredients well. Add the diced tomatoes and chicken in the pan and stir well. Adjust the salt and paper according to your taste.

Now pour in the chicken broth, orange juice, flaxseed, oregano and allow the mixture to come to boil. When the mixture is reduced to half take it out in a bowl and serve with your favorite tacos.

Tacos with Chicken and Pineapple

Serving: 4 Persons

Cooking Time: 1 hour 40 minutes

Ingredients:

4 taco shells (Hard or soft according to your choice)

0.5 kg of skinless boneless chicken breast, cut into chunks

1 cup of green bell pepper, chopped

1 cup of onion, chopped

0.5 kg pineapples cubes

2 tablespoon of cooking fat

Sea salt to taste

Pepper to taste

Process:

Place a pan on the stove and add the oil in the pan. Add the chicken and sauté it in the oil until the chicken is cooked and tender. When the chicken is cooked, take it out and add the pineapples in the same pan. Sauté them in the remnant oil for 2-3 minutes now and the rest of the vegetables and cook them until they are cooked.

Add the chicken in the pan and sauté all the ingredients together. Adjust the salt and pepper and serve it with hard shelled tacos.

Tacos with green Chicken Tikka

Serving: 10 Persons

Cooking Time: 1.5 hours

Ingredients:

5-6 taco shells (soft or hard)

2 tablespoon of red chili powder

3 tablespoon of green chilies (chopped coarsely)

3 tablespoon of parsley (chopped coarsely)

1 tablespoon of grass fed butter

1 tablespoon of Mustard Powder

1 tablespoon of oregano crushed

2 bunches Coriander leaves

1.5 tablespoon of balsamic vinegar

2 Tablespoon of coconut flour

2 tablespoon of flaxseed meal

4tablespoon of coconut milk

Salt to taste

Pepper to taste

Turmeric powder, half teaspoon

Half teaspoon of nutmeg powder

3 tablespoon olive oil

1 kg of chicken boneless, cut into cubes

Process:

Take a large bowl and add all the ingredients in it except taco shell. (red chili powder, green chilies, parsley, butter, Mustard Powder, oregano, Coriander leaves, vinegar coconut flour, flaxseed meal, coconut milk, Salt to taste, Pepper to taste, Turmeric powder, nutmeg powder, olive oil and chicken). Mix all the ingredients together and place aside to marinade the chicken for approx 1 hour. Now take pan and pour in 2-3 tablespoon of oil and the chicken with all the mixture in the pan and mix well and Sauté the chicken and the mixture over high flame for 5 minutes. Turn the flame down to medium. Add half cup of water and place a lid on the pan and allow the chicken to get tender.

When ready take the chicken Tikka off of the skewers and place them on taco shells. Serve immediately.

Tacos with Shrimp and fruit salsa

Serving: 4 Persons

Cooking Time: 25 Minutes

Ingredients:

4 taco shells (Hard or soft according to your choice)

1 Kg raw shrimp, (cleaned and deshelled)

2 cups of mangoes, cut into cubes

1 cup apple cut into cubes

1 cup of orange cut into pieces (deseeded)

1 cup cranberries

1 cup avocado, cut into thin slices

1 tablespoon of lime juice

Olive oil (according to need)

Sea salt to taste

Black pepper to taste

Process:

Take a bowl and add all the fruits in it and add lemon juice and mix well. In the meanwhile, take a pan and add olive oil in it. Add the shrimp once the oil in hot and sauté them for 1 minute. Sprinkle the salt and pepper from top and sauté some more.

When the prawns are a bit golden take them out. Cut the prawns into 2-3 pieces and add the pieces in the fruit mixture. Mix well and serve with your favorite taco.

Tacos with Oven Omelet

Serving: 4 People

Cooking Time: 20 Minutes

Ingredients:

5-6 taco shells (soft or hard)

6 eggs (whisked)

Half a cup of coconut milk

0.25 cup mushrooms, cut into slices

0.25 cup bell pepper, cut into slices

0.25 cup onions cut into slices

1 tablespoon of chives, coarsely chopped

Black pepper to taste

Sea salt to taste

Process:

Heat the oven at 350F. Take a bowl and pour in milk and whisked eggs. Adjust the salt and pepper. Take a pizza baking dish. Grease it with olive oil. Pour in the egg mixture and add the rest of the ingredients from top ad stir a bit.

Place the dish in the oven and bake for 10 minutes or until cooked. Serve with your favorite taco.

Tacos with Salmon salad

Serving: 10-12 Persons

Cooking Time: 30 Minutes

Ingredients:

10-12 Tacos

0.5 Kg salmon, strips

3 tablespoon Olive oil

Sea salt & Pepper to taste

3 cups of broccoli florets (boiled)

4 cups of salad greens

2 cups of lettuce

Half a cup of capsicum, Juliana cut

1 cup onion, slices

Process:

Take a bowl and add strips of salmon in it. Season it with salt and pepper. In the meanwhile, take a pan and heat oil in it. Add the salmon and brown it. Add all the vegetables in a bowl and toss them together.

Now add the strips of salmon in the bowl and mix well. Place the mixture in taco of your choice and serve.

Tacos with Turkey, Avocado and Spinach

Serving: 8-10 Persons

Cooking Time: 25 Minutes

Ingredients:

10-12 Tacos

1 Kg Boneless turkey (strips)

1.5 cup of avocado (cubes)

1 teaspoon of garlic, chopped

1 cup red bell pepper, (cubes)

1 cup of spinach, (chopped)

Half cup of green onions, chopped

6 tablespoon of avocado oil

2 tablespoon of lemon juice

Sea salt & Pepper, to taste

Process:

In a skillet and add olive oil. Add garlic and sauté until fragrant. Add the turkey in the skillet and stir. Cook the turkey cubes until tender.

Add the capsicum and spinach in skillet and stir well. Adjust the seasoning according to your taste. Take out the turkey, spinach and capsicum and add oil in the skillet. Add the avocados, green onions; lemon juice and sauté them. Cook the vegetables for 3-4 minutes and then add the turkey in the skillet. Mix well and Serve with the tacos shell of your choice.

Tacos with Sweet potato salad

Serving: 5-6 Persons

Cooking Time: 2 Hour

Ingredients:

5-6 hard Shell tacos

1 cup of mushrooms, (sliced)

1 cup boiled sweet potato cut into small cubes

0.5 kg chicken (strips)

1 cup coconut milk;

1 cup of green collards (boiled),

0.5 cup balsamic vinegar

1 teaspoon of grounded mustard powder

5-6 Tablespoon of Avocado Oil

Sea salt to taste

Pepper to taste

Process:

In a bowl add chicken in it. Adjust the salt and pepper. In another pan heat oil and add the chicken strips and brown them. Add green collards and other vegetables and sauté them for 5 minutes. Add the balsamic vinegar and allow the mixture to come to boil

Place a lid and cook to allow the chicken to get tender. When all the liquid in the pan gets dried, let the sauce get a bit thick, check for seasoning. In another pan add 1 tablespoon of oil and then add the sweet potatoes. And fry them a bit. Add the sweet potatoes in the pan and stir. Place the chicken and a bit of sauce in the taco shells and serve immediately.

Taco with a slice of meat loaf

Serving: 10 Persons

Cooking Time: 2 hours

Ingredients:

10-12 Tacos

1 kg beef (grounded)

1 tablespoon of sea salt

1 tablespoon of black pepper

1 egg (whisked)

1 cup of onion, chopped

2 cups of button mushrooms, finely chopped

1 tablespoon of chili pepper flakes

1.5 tablespoon of thyme, minced

1 tablespoon of fresh oregano, crushed

3 cloves of garlic, crushed

½ cup homemade ketchup

1 tablespoon of raw honey

½ tablespoon of Worcestershire sauce

1 tablespoon of Olive oil

Process:

Heat the oven at 350 F. In the meanwhile take a skillet and place it on flame. Add oil and sauté mushrooms in it. Allow the mushrooms to get a bit soft. In the meanwhile, mix salt, pepper, thyme, oregano, chilies and crushed garlic together. Add the meat in the bowl and mix the spices with the meat loaf. Now add the glazed mushrooms in the bowl and mix them well. Add raw honey and ketchup and mix them well.

Now take a loaf pan and grease it with olive oil. Transfer the meat mixture in the pan and place the baking pan inside the preheated oven. Bake the meat loaf for about 40 minutes. Take the loaf out and allow it to cool down a bit. Take the loaf and cut it into slice. Serve with the soft shelled taco or cut it into chunks to be served with hard shelled tacos.

Tacos with Melon Salsa

Serving: 5 Persons

Cooking Time: 20 Minutes

Ingredients:

5 Tacos (hard or soft shell, according to your choice)

1 cup of watermelon, cut into cubes

1 cup of cantaloupe, cut into cubes

1 cup of honeydew melon, cut into cubes

Half cup of cucumbers, seeded and cut into cubes

0.25 cup of red onion, cut into cubes

0.25 cup of avocado, chopped

2 tablespoon of cilantro, coarsely chopped

5 tablespoon of lime juice

Sea salt to taste

Freshly ground pepper to taste

Process:

Take a bowl and add all the vegetables and fruits (watermelon, cantaloupe, melon, cucumbers, avocado and onion) in it except for the taco shells. Mix all the fruits and vegetables together and sprinkle salt, pepper and cilantro and mix well. Drizzle the honey and mix with help of spoon. Fill the taco shells generously and serve. Enjoy!

Tacos with Fish Fillet and Pepper Salsa

Serving: Serves 4

Cooking Time: 30 Minutes

Ingredients:

1 cup of water

1 tsp lemon zest

1/2 bunch fresh and minced mint leaves

2 pounds sole fillets (or your favorite white fish)

2 red bell peppers, chopped

2 tbsp Dijon or homemade mustard

2 tbsp lemon juice

4 tbsp extra-virgin olive oil

Process:

Take a large pan and add the oil in the pan. When the oil is ready, add red bell peppers in the pan and sauté them over medium heat. In the meanwhile take a bowl and add the mustard, olive oil, lemon juice and zest, mint and the seated bell peppers and mix well and put the bowl aside.

Heat a pan and grease the pan with Paleo oil (Olive or Avocado oil preferably) and place the salmon fillet in the pan and grill it form each side for 2-3 minutes before changing the sides.

Take the fish out of the pan and place it in a platter and add water in the pan and scrap the pan to dissolve the flavor form the pan in water. Now add the bell pepper mixture in the pan and stir well. When the sauce is a bit thick, cut the salmon fillet into strips and add them to pan. Gently roll them to cover them in sauce. Serve with your favorite taco shells.

Tacos with Chicken and Herbs

__Serving:__ 8 persons

__Cooking Time:__ 1 Hour

__Ingredients__:

8 Taco shells (hard or soft tacos shells of your choice)

2 pounds of minced chicken

0.5 cup of green onions, chopped

0.5 cup of almond flour

1 egg, (whisked)

1 teaspoon of chili powder

Olive oil

Pepper and Salt according to taste

2 tablespoon of balsamic vinegar

1 cup homemade ketchup puree

0.5 cup of finely chopped onion

0.5 tablespoon of paprika

2 tablespoon of coconut aminos

__Process:__

Heat an oven at 400F. In a bowl mix all the ingredients other than of the sauce. Mix chicken, almond flour, green onions, whisked eggs and chili powder the ingredients and knead them to make it one.

If the mixture gets a bit dry, add 2-3 tablespoon of olive oil and knead again. Then take the mixture and form small crocket. Place them aside. Take baking tray grease it with oil, place the crockets on the try and place the tray in the pre heated oven.

In the mean while prepare the sauce for the chicken crockets. Take a large skillet and add olive oil heat it up and then add homemade ketchup and stir well. Adjust the salt and pepper and pour in the balsamic vinegar. Add the onions coconut aminos and paprika in the pan and stir well. Heat until the consistency of the sauce is a bit thick.

Take out the crockets from the oven and add them to the sauce. Stir well make sure you don't break the crockets. Now take the tacos and add crockets in the center with the BBQ sauce and roll it. Secure with tooth pick. Serve hot.

Tacos with Salmon Sauce and Banana

**Serving:** 5 Persons

**Cooking Time:** 40 Minutes

**Ingredients:**

5 Taco shells (soft or hard according to your choice)

5 Salmon fillets (Medium sized)

Olive oil

1 cup of coconut milk

1 tablespoon of red curry paste (homemade)

3 tablespoon of lemon juice

3 green onions, thinly sliced

1 cup of bananas, cut into thick slices

2 tablespoon of slivered almonds

Half a cup of chopped cilantro

Sea salt to taste

Pepper to taste

**Process:**

Take the salmon fillets in a tray and sprinkle the lemon zest and lemon juice on top. Apply them all over the fillet and rub well. Sprinkle the salt and pepper and rub it all over the filets.

Place a pan on the stove and add 2-3 tablespoon of oil in the pan and add the fillets in the pan. Don't over crowd it, leave enough space to move the fillets. Grill the fish from both sides on medium flame. When the crust becomes a bit golden brown take the fillet out of the pan.

In another pan heat oil and add the red curry paste and sauté. When fragrant, add the green pinions, cilantro and bananas in the pan. Sauté them well. Stir in the almonds and add a little water and cook for 3 minutes with lid on. Cut the salmon fillet into stripes and add it into the sauce. Stir gently. Serve with your favorite type of taco shells.

Conclusion

Paleo diet refers to the Paleolithic diet pattern that existed long before we opted for relatively unhealthy lifestyle. This diet has its own perks. Paleo diet may appear unappealing due to its omission of some ingredients. But if you know how to cook your favorite food the Paleo way you will start to appreciate the changes this diet can bring in your health. Try out these scrumptious Paleo Taco recipes and let us know how it worked out for you.